HOW TO SURVIVE PSYCHOSIS

HOW TO SURVIVE PSYCHOSIS

POPPY ATKINS

Poppy Atkins

Contents

To my mum for always being there for me through terribly hard times. To Jane for your cover art. To Robyn and Jack for attempting to understand your very confusing sister over the years; for your support and love in adulthood. To dad, David and Josie for being close and supportive over my lifetime. To my nieces and nephew, Frankie, Eleanor, Emilia and Digby, may you draw inspiration and education from this book. To my friends for sticking it out. To my editor Caitilin at Artful Words, your support and knowledge has been amazing. To my doctors and psychologists that have read and supported this work. To my students and colleagues, thank you for trying to make sense of me at times I couldn't.

First Printing, 2024

Foreword

Hello!

As a person afflicted with a chronic illness, I always want people to know I am more than that. Because of my own internal prejudices, I have sometimes written off all the details of my identity and just said to myself, 'I'm schizophrenic; that's all there is to me.' Sometimes I have felt that that's what others would think of me if they knew. But I have a whole complex personality and rich preferences for things that I love and dislike. I have a great many friends, and I have a myriad of faults. I am still uncertain about identifying as having a disability. It's all very tricky. I don't even really know about the medical model and social model of disability in terms of how they apply to me. I know I currently can't talk about my illness or tell my work about it. I know there is still a huge stigma. But I also know that I need to write this book to tell you how I deal with my psychosis in the hope that it might help you or someone you know.

Psychosis is something I have lived with since I was 20. I might be called schizophrenic, although I don't have auditory or visual hallucinations. Instead, I get intense and detailed delusions. These are catastrophic in terms of living a stable life. I have had many psychoses over the years, and they always leave me picking up both the mental and physical pieces they leave behind. I have had to pay back debts, settle into new towns and houses, and reframe my thinking about so many things that I was convinced were real. In terms of my life trajectory, I have been so busy surviving psychosis that I have missed out on key life events and lessons. I have chosen not to have children because of my illness, and I do not have a partner, which adds some challenges but also frees me up to do the things I love on my terms.

I often tell people how bad it was "then" and how good it is now—when I *am* good, that is. I trick myself into thinking that this time, *this* time, was the last time. If I change my living arrangements and my job, if I move away from family, if I move closer to family, if I go on adventures more often, if I live in a smaller house, once I buy a house, when I finally settle down, these things might alleviate or even prevent the next psychosis. It might be a bookend in my life. My life might be psychosis-free one day, and I will be cured. What a dream! And every time a psychosis happens, I find ways to believe it won't happen again. I get the idea that there is an ending to it. A finale. But I am getting older now, and my life has gone in cycles that I can now see quite clearly.

The cycle for me goes like this: I am fine and happy, a bit overweight, taking my meds. Then I get stressed or something happens, I put on weight or break up with someone. I think I need to move towns or jobs. Then I get psychosis, lose weight, cut people out of my life and stop talking. I move towns or jobs, then at some point I realise I need help and I get it, then I am fine and happy again. Rinse and repeat. This has happened to me over the course of my twenties and thirties and has left me with not much savings and starting a new job yet again. However, I am about to turn 40, and I want to capitalise on my strengths. I have a home and career, I am going to finish my second master's degree, and people generally like me. I am in a place in my life where I can reflect and give advice on psychosis. I am gratefully recovering from schizophrenia, and I think I am in the right place to help others.

I called this book *How to Survive Psychosis* because it's a collection of my experiences and survival tools. I would like to note here that this is not medical or professional advice. These are things that have worked for me over a long period of time, and they are things I wish I had known about when I was first experiencing psychosis. I refer to life with psychosis as "coasting the psychosis" or living with it. It's not about "surviving and thriving" because psychosis is chronic and relentless. I would love to be surviving and thriving, and in some ways I am, but psychosis is something I am going to have to deal with forever. This has been a sobering realisation as I come into middle age.

I use the terms "schizophrenia" and "psychosis" inter-changeably in this book, as my exact diagnosis is still to be determined, and labels are not always helpful for people. What I do know is that I suffer from wild, grandiose and persecutory delusions regularly and go through cycles of depression and acceptance that see me making big, life-changing decisions. I make these decisions to try to alleviate the experience of psychosis, and they are tied in with my denial and deep hopes it won't happen again. I feel great shame that I am "different" and experience these strange things that other people do not. I want so desperately to be like everyone else, and that is why I have such denial and hope. I desperately want to belong. My illness is debilitating and confusing, and it leaves me feeling hopeless and "less than." This feeling comes both from within me and from the way people who know about my illness respond when I have been in a psychosis. My friends and family treat me like I am sick, like there is something wrong with me and I am in need of help. Usually, my denial kicks in and I think they are patronising me.

I also have low self-esteem because this has been happening to me for nearly twenty years, and I have a belief that I am different and kind of broken. I think people see me as sick and a victim to the illness, and when I see myself like that, I have a big cry. It's not always like that, though. When I am well and things are going smoothly, I can reflect and feel so grateful for the things I have achieved and done in my "abnormal" life. I am also fiercely resilient, constantly making meaning and questioning things in my identity. I have had to come up with solutions out of necessity because of this illness, and somehow in the midst of the shame about being different, I also believe I am capable. This is one thing that has saved me and allowed me to have a career and relative success amid the mess that is schizophrenia: holding onto that tiny shred of confidence.

I am writing this book because I see myself as someone who has survived and is surviving psychosis. I want to help other people who suffer from it. I want to be an advocate for people who live with complex mental health, and I want to share what has worked for me in my 20 years' experience of schizophrenia. I want to tell my story so others can relate to it and take from it what they want, using any of the things that I found worked for me. I want to contribute to what might be a newer social model of mental health and to create a community where it is okay to talk about and be proud of what we live through. In such a community, it might be that working all the time is not valued as highly as looking after your health. It might mean living in a less capitalistic society where values are more important than profits, which could be beneficial not just for those experiencing mental illness. I want to foster an understanding of schizophrenia and to break down stigma. I want to share what has and has not worked for me and to make my experience meaningful, both for myself and for you who is reading this.

Chapter 1

Tell someone

I am riding my bike to the supermarket to get some soy milk, and my mind is going a thousand miles an hour. Who made this milk? Was it made in China? How much carbon did it take to make? Do I deserve to purchase and consume such a product? I am a waste of oxygen. I am a contributor to the demise of the environment. I am the cause of climate change. It is all my fault, and everyone knows. Everyone knows something about me. There are people spying on me, wanting me to die. I deserve to die because I have caused climate change.

My first piece of advice for when you might be experiencing something strange in your mind—like if you now think something in your life means something different or has a special significance that it didn't used to, for example—is to tell someone. You might think that you need to die because of an obscure reason, or you might think that you are to blame for something like climate change: it could be any number of things. Tell someone. Tell a trusted friend, tell your parents, tell your counsellor or your doctor. Get help. You need to talk about what is going on. If you are thinking things that are different or suspect you are hearing or seeing things that no one else can, you must reach out. You need to get help, get out of your head and connect with someone who might be able to help you or give you some advice. You need to be open to this. People close to you might have noticed you are behaving differently or seen your mood change. If it is feeling weird inside your mind, like things are not making sense, *tell someone.*

When I had my first psychosis, I thought the fly in my room had a camera in it and that people could read my mind. My most recent brief psychosis saw me thinking that my boss could read my mind and get into it and give me messages. You need to tell someone if something like this is happening to you. It makes it so much worse if you keep it all in, and it gets worse if you don't get help early. The delusions get more ingrained and harder to get out of. You start to believe them more than you believe the people on the outside. Make an appointment with a medical professional, tell your friend what you are thinking or seeing or hearing, put it into the world, because that's the only way you're going to get support and try to get better.

I say this and it sounds easy, but it's not as easy as you might think. You first need to understand that what you are thinking is not real, and this can be really hard. I didn't understand what was going on during my first psychosis, and this continued to be the biggest challenge in all my psychoses. I believed what was happening. I really thought the world was blaming me for global warming, and I thought drowning myself in the ocean was the only answer. The build-up to this was a long one. I couldn't sleep. I thought people were spying on me and that they were in a secret plan to find me guilty of environmental crimes. I thought all my friends at university knew something I didn't. I acted quiet, and my flatmates asked me if anything was wrong. Of course, I was still at the age where fitting in was everything, so I said, 'Nothing, all good.'

Back then, being sick was seen as a weakness, both in my family and in society. Mental illness was still taboo. I was petrified of being seen as someone who was "sick," "less than," "faulty" or different. I could not stand to be classed as anything but cool and fun, which I tried so hard to be. I thought drinking alcohol and partying was a way to make friends and find a sense of belonging that was hugely important to me.

But I was stressed. I had been elected to the student council and I was studying drama. These were really public things to be doing in the university community. I was also drinking excessively very frequently. I was smoking pot and not getting enough sleep. The student council election and the drama studies were big things for me, and I couldn't cope with them. I wasn't ready to take a political stance, and I wasn't confident enough to be an actor. There was a conspiracy going on with everyone. Everything seemed to have a deeper meaning. The student council was using me as a political football because I wasn't completely sure of my opinions. The groups we were put in for drama performances were a secret plan by the lecturer to teach me I was actually a terrible person. I was flipping out, like sometimes happened when I smoked marijuana. I panicked and felt awful. I didn't know what was going on, what was real and what was happening to me, and this was happening all the time, even when I wasn't under the influence.

I made an appointment to see the university counsellor because I thought I could sort out all the things that were getting on top of me, including the conspiracies. I held off telling anyone anything that was going on behind my eyes until the day of the appointment. I got into the lift to go up to the student services office, and in the mirror inside the lift I saw I had a pimple bleeding near my mouth. I processed this in my mind to mean I had been sucking people's blood like the demon I was. I got into the counsellor's office and told them in truncated sentences that I thought people were spying on me and I needed to kill myself. I remember the counsellor telling me that I needed to go to the hospital, so we made a plan. I would ride my bike home, ask one of my flatmates to drive me to the hospital, and then tell the doctors there what was happening. And I did exactly that.

The fact I told these things to that counsellor led to a two-week hospitalisation, during which I battled with what was real and what wasn't. My friends and family came to visit me, and I was severely anxious about my identity now that I was "mentally unwell" to them. I talked with psychiatrists and psychologists and was assigned a caseworker when I got out of hospital. I went on medication, and I adjusted to this "thing" that had happened to me. I got support from my family and friends, and I felt cared for. There was no diagnosis at that time except that I had had a psychotic episode. I didn't think it would happen again. I would get better and still have a good life. I would recover. This was just a one-off, and I could take the medication until I got better and then leave this behind me. It was a hard adjustment for me from being "normal" and "okay" to being "mentally unwell." I didn't want to accept this as a part of me (and I never have). So, being Poppy who went to hospital for two weeks because she went "crazy" was huge for me to deal with in a pretty public community at university.

Telling people when I am getting sick has never been easy. There are a few factors involved in this. One is that I am believing in the delusions; for example, if I believe that my mum is actually evil, then I don't reach out to her. Another is that I am afraid of being a burden and getting sick again, that all the hard work I did in getting well will be undone if I admit what is happening, and that people at work might find out or I might lose my job. This is a lot to deal with when you believe you're being spied on or that a conspiracy about the world is coming to you as a special message on the television.

In order to tell people you are getting sick, you need to have insight that things are going wrong in your mind, and you need to believe that people will help you and that you are worthy of help. I know I have refused help from friends and loved ones on many occasions out of denial that anything is wrong. I have even gone to the doctor to appease my mum, only to get in there and lie, saying my symptoms weren't as bad as they really were. All this comes from fear of being seen as dependent on others, fear of being told that there is something wrong with me. All the shame I have around being different or having something faulty in me really comes out when I am sick. My mum and family have had to wait, power-less, many times until I come to the conclusion that I need help. This is usually after I have made huge financial decisions or created a big mess in my life.

I think that that first appointment with the counsellor at university was pivotal, though. My description of what was going on, when put into the world verbally and heard by someone else, set the wheels in motion for me to get help. It began a lifetime of my being able to see psychosis as something that was happening to me but wasn't *actually me*. It was where my insight, which has gotten better over time, began. It also made me realise that this happens to other people, there's a name for it and that I wasn't alone. My family still loved me. My friends still cared for me.

I was told time and again, and I eventually realised, that experiencing psychosis is like having a cold or a broken leg, only it is mental. But mental illness is shrouded by stigma and shame because you don't "look" sick. Some people can't understand illness if there is no physical appearance of being unwell. Fortunately, mental health awareness has come a long way since my first experience of psychosis in 2005. Organisations such as SANE Australia, the Black Dog Institute and Beyond Blue have created more safety around discussing mental health, and it has become more socially acceptable to have a mental illness. People "coming out" on social media and explaining their experience, advances in the social model of disability, and changes to mental health care have all been pivotal in how things are different, today.

'Tangle'
They took my knitting needles from me,
The wool knotted, like my thoughts,
Committed.

The first psychosis of many,
Patchwork delusions, identity,
Obliterated.

Schizophrenia, a mosaic
Of years and ideas—internal,
Attended.

Life-changing medication
And support like crochet stitching,
Connected.

Today, meaning is more stable,
Like a leadlight window,
Reflected.

Chapter 2

Take your meds

The next point of advice I have that has worked for me is to take your meds. Get a doctor's appointment, get a prescription, go to the pharmacy, fill the prescription, and take the medication as directed. Again, like the advice in the last chapter, this is easier said than done.

When I went to the psych ward that first time, I was prescribed medication, and I took it for about six months. This saw me come back to reality, and the delusions went away. I was able to finish the semester of university and keep moving through life as I wanted. My 21st birthday occurred, and I planned an overseas trip. It was all very exciting, except I was putting on a lot of weight. I had to buy bigger clothes, and I felt ashamed. I was hungry all the time, which was one of the side effects of the medication.

I'd love to write here that I went on proudly in my new body, but I was a young women brought up under the patriarchy where being thin is valued, and I had definitely had my share of disordered eating and diets up till then (and for many years later). So, instead of embracing who I was and how I looked, I turned against the medication. I wanted to be thin, so I stopped taking the meds and started jogging. This, I thought, would be the cure. If I got fit enough, I would never have a psychosis again. Surely! I would be successful if I was thin, and mental illness would simply go away because I was fine again.

I jogged and jogged. I also played soccer at university with my friends in a team called the Hippos. It was so much fun. We had a beautiful bunch of girls, with many of us only just learning the game but having a ripper of a time socially while getting fit. I got so fit and improved so much at playing soccer that I won the coach's award. This was great for me; I love tangible achievement. I felt so proud. I was a size 8 and thought I was so hot and attractive to all the guys and girls. I was absolutely high on the rush of finally achieving something big, something everyone could see, something I could be really proud of. This was overshadowed by my heavy drinking and promiscuity that my friends saw, but they didn't say anything to me about it. I was a force to be reckoned with. I thought I was well, and I thought I had conquered my illness. I was actually going to be a success.

Like all good things, this time ended, and I fell into another psychosis. I began crying all the time and thinking things had deeper meanings. My friends and I were on a winery walkabout in Albury, and I couldn't stop crying because a guy on the bus was pretending to drink cleaning product. What was the message behind this? What was he *really* trying to tell me? I could not see past it. I was quiet and withdrawn. I kept crying, and my friends thought they should leave me in Albury to be with my mum. I was so mortified. This was failure; I was failing again. I was less than, not good enough, "sick" and broken.

I went back into denial and I got angry. I was angry at myself, angry that this was happening to me, and angry about how unfair it all was. It was so difficult to deal with social views of being sick and my own inner prejudice about having a mental illness. I really thought being crazy meant you were a social outcast. I felt like I didn't belong and that I would never be accepted by society with this illness. The outlook for my future was grim. I felt awful shame and I wanted to die.

Mum took me to the hospital, where they prescribed medication for me again. I spoke to the doctor, but I was difficult to deal with and blamed everyone else for thinking something was wrong. If I had hidden it better, then nothing would be wrong. I also blamed myself for being such a loser and not having everything together like everyone else. I didn't want to put the weight back on, and I didn't want to be seen as a failure after everything I had just achieved. My anger was red hot, and I felt so powerless. I thought everyone was trying to bring me down. The fact they had noticed something meant something really was wrong. I hadn't been able to hide it well enough. The anger was not helpful at this time because it made me lash out. It made me wild.

I left the hospital with a packet of some different antipsychotics. Livid, I didn't speak to anyone in the family home. I went to my room and lay down, crying. I was so furious I swallowed the whole packet of medicine that night. My mum and sister found me, and I was rushed to the hospital in the back of the family car. I was barely conscious. At the hospital, they pumped my stomach, and I went in and out of consciousness for a few days. It was my sister's birthday, and I had ruined it. I had also broken a very important rule: to take your medication exactly as prescribed. It took me years to regain my doctors' trust to prescribe me whole packets of medication because I always mentioned I had overdosed. I was scared for myself. It wasn't a temptation, rather I just couldn't predict my behaviour. My life seemed so messy and horrible, and going back over my story again and again with doctors was difficult.

Take your meds. I have had prolonged periods of stability when I have taken my medication. This, I am so grateful for. In these times, I have completed three degrees, almost finishing my fourth, built a career, saved money, and maintained friendships and relationships. I have lived in many places and gained great experience. I have always been fortunate enough to be able to afford my medication, and I know many people can't. Thank god for the Pharmaceutical Benefits Scheme in Australia and the fact that I have always managed to hold down a job. People with schizophrenia are often homeless and live in poverty. I see them in Melbourne, talking to themselves on Swanston Street, and I know I was once like them, only I didn't make it to homelessness. I feel so grateful that I kept a roof over my head and have been able to support myself. This, I believe, is only because I have complied with what doctors have told me to do, and one of these things is taking my meds.

It has taken me lots of stopping and starting with different medications to find one that works for me, and even now there is a plethora of side effects that I live with. Side effects are a huge part of why people don't take their medication. I have been so fortunate that the side effects of my medication haven't been too bad for me. I still put on weight and eat a lot. This is something I battle with every day. I have high levels of prolactin, which means I can't have kids and have osteoporosis. I am hungry nearly all the time. I have had numerous discussions with loved ones and doctors about the compromise between side effects and the benefit for mental health that I get from these medicines. Not having children isn't something that was stolen from me by the medication, but it has been a big part of my consideration when thinking about whether or not to become a mum. My weight is something I always battle with, but again, society is changing and not being stick thin is okay these days.

For me, these side effects contrast with the disaster that is psychosis. I have personally weighed up the benefits of being able to keep a sound mind against the side effects I get when taking medication. The side effects have been less dramatic for my life holistically than if I am not on meds. I have learnt, over many years, that my episodes are fewer and occur to a lesser degree when I take my medication. It is not a cure, I know, but I am more stable on them. My two most recent psychoses have been quite brief, and I have had insight to take a few days off work and go to the doctor. But it is never neat and tidy.

I had a prolonged psychosis in my thirties that lasted five months because I wasn't taking my meds. Again, I wanted to lose weight after a dreamboat of a guy I dated told me I needed to. Everything had been going well for me for a long time due to taking my meds, and I began to think I could do without them. That psychosis was the worst to date. It was a terrible time in my life when I thought I was the Queen of Australia, and I went $30,000 in debt to buy a campervan to run away from an impending war. The TV was talking directly to me, and I shunned all my family, who I thought were bringing me down because I was the secret Queen, meaning that it was known only by a few special, powerful men and I had to be protected and worshipped. My family did not believe I was the Queen, therefore I had to shun them. I was so sick that I went into the classroom in which I was supposed to be teaching and played videos for the students because I was incapable of giving the lesson. I went quiet, and my colleagues knew something was wrong. I

bought lipstick and jewellery with a personal loan because the Queen deserved free money. I shaved my head
because I got the message to do so through the kitchen
window from my otherwise innocuous neighbours.

It was all so shocking and dramatic yet also so slow and
insidious that it seemed okay. I don't know why that is,
and I can't explain how it all seems to make sense when
you're in the middle of it. It just seems logical when it is
happening. It's kind of like I think things, then make up
a meaning for them, then believe it. Then I add to each
thought a reason why it's all happening. I wasn't able to
access another perspective, I was extremely alone, and
my mind went on its own into a dreamland that I could
not escape from. There was an excitement in having this
"knowledge" about my status. I got a lot of dopamine
(which is characteristic of schizophrenia) from thinking
I was the Queen. It made me feel special and thrilled.
Looking back on this time, I want to hug the little lonely
girl in her beach shack who was shaving her head and
sleeping in a van outside. This psychosis concluded with
me moving as close to Albury as I could get, finding a
community psychiatrist, and going on a high dose of a
new medication that I am still on today.

It has taken years to really understand and acknowl-
edge how important medication is for me. Sometimes I
question how much time I have wasted by going off my
medication and the subsequent disaster the psychosis
leaves me in, which makes me sad. I feel silly and like I
am not good enough, especially when all my friends and

family live lives that are moving onwards and upwards. Those instances have required so much money to pay back debts, buy new cars, and move towns over and over to get myself back on some kind of track. But over time, I have learnt to accept this is a part of my journey, and I accept that life in general is hard and full of disappointment. I understand things aren't perfect and everyone has their own issues. Truly, I have been chasing the cure for so long, but I have had to conclude that there isn't one. This has been harrowing for me. I wanted to get better and see my life play out in a successful way. I wanted to be normal and be seen as normal. There is no cure, though. This, I have to accept.

In the past, I wanted to be thin and be seen as successful for that, but I have had to accept that this may never be the case for me. I have had to adjust what success means to me. I used to think marriage and a family and a home was success, but I don't have that either. I believe my success comes through living relatively well with schizophrenia. I have wanted to be psychosis-free, seeing an end to the tumult that occurs when I have an episode, but I have to accept that this is not a reality for me. Things aren't perfect. Life is full of disappointment, but I count my blessings. I do all of this, but first, I take my medication day and night. (There might also be a lesson about body image in there for me to learn, too.)

Medication should be taken as prescribed, and you should be very honest about this with your psychiatrist or doctor. It might take a few goes to get the right dose and type of medication for you, and it is important to recognise that they work slowly and work well for *some* people. They do not work for everyone. This is a reality. But trying them and finding one that works can be life-changing. I am truly humbled by how they have helped me to have normal thoughts that I can live a day-to-day life with. I still have to do a lot of therapy and work to forget or counter the beliefs I built in psychosis, but the medication, for me, has helped dramatically. I recommend giving it a try if you have psychosis.

'Relearn'
I've had to relearn meaning
Post-psychosis.
Undo all the knots and mazes
Of things I thought were real.
Back in it, I drowned in fabrication,
My mind the boss.
Unknown cues and nuance
At work, on TV
All added up to:
"It's all about me."
Me as special and powerful,
Me as the secret Queen.
A noise with deeper
Significance,
In psychosis nothing's just
By chance.
Innocuous doesn't exist,

Everything intense.
I've had to relearn meaning.

Chapter 3

Get a team around you and keep your appointments

Doctor Smith knows things aren't alright for me. I am off work and going to his office to get checked up and get a medical certificate. I am hiding the fact that I have written in permanent marker all over the wall at my rental the names of the people who are going to die because they don't believe I am the secret Queen of Australia. Doctor Smith is gentle and takes my blood pressure. He suggests going to see a psychiatrist. He says he just wants me to get better. I believe him. Something in me trusts him. I need to do what he says. I need to get things back to normal. I realise that things aren't normal.

The next point of advice I will give anyone going through psychosis is to get a team around you and keep your appointments with them. Find a general practitioner, psychiatrist, psychologist, dietitian (if necessary), support worker, counsellor, and friends and family to wrap around you and keep you accountable. Accountability is important because it keeps you connected. It's so easy to get caught up in your own internal world in psychosis, so keeping accountable to others helps immensely with this. You aren't an island, so don't isolate yourself from those who can support and care for you. The people I have wrapped around me over time are there to help me and to go in and bat for me when I need it. You need people like this around you too. Keep your appointments and meet-ups with these people. Be honest with them because they are there for you! Tell them exactly what is happening. Masking and hiding what's going on does not help anyone understand your situation. They are left confused and will make up their own minds about what's happening, and this is not helpful. Honesty, in contrast, is liberating and conducive to solutions. It might be hard to be honest with those around you, but trust me, it is better than believing what is happening in your mind!

Like the other advice in this book, it has been hard for me to do this because telling people the truth felt like I was admitting defeat, that I was failing. There was so much fear around telling my team when I needed help. I wanted so badly to be okay, so I would often mask and hide. But later in my life, I found that telling people about my strange thoughts stops me believing them because we can all see they are ridiculous. The more people I have that I can call on the phone when I need to talk, the better it is for me. Get a team like this for yourself, and turn up to all your appointments so you can get the help you deserve. Over the years, I found it difficult to believe I deserved help because I was so busy blaming myself for the psychosis. I thought it was a defect in my whole self, but that isn't true for me, and it's not true for you either. Sometimes I thought nothing would help me, but help is out there, and you have to find a way to get to a point where you believe that.

I have been in some pretty horrible psychoses, and what helped me out of them was turning up to every appointment and telling the practitioner what was happening. But this wasn't always the case. So many times, I lied about my symptoms or angrily stayed quiet. I often didn't have the insight at the time, or I was too full of shame that I was sick. I regret how I was during these visits to specialists and doctors because I could have been treated quicker and gotten into less of a mess if I had been more honest. This is so vital to getting better.

At the appointment when I got a diagnosis of schizophrenia, I hardly said a word. The report said the doctor could not tell whether there was any internal stimuli and they had to go on what my family members had said. I sat in the room thinking it was all part of my evil mother's plan to lock me back up in hospital. I was cajoled by my GP, whom I trusted, to go to this appointment, and I drove there with the radio talking directly to me. My initial impressions were that the psychiatrist's office was calm and clean and expensive, and I didn't like it. I was signing my life away and my death was imminent, or so I thought. Even though I didn't really do or say much during the appointment, I got a diagnosis, which gave me a label. They say that to name something is to tame it, but I wasn't sure about anything by then. It was another case of moving home and trying to make sense of what had happened, after I began taking the new prescription of antipsychotics.

This process of making sense of everything that has happened is another part of that cycle of psychosis I go through, and it's an important way that I have involved my team. Using your team to help you make sense of things gives everyone a shared explanation of what happened in the psychosis and an understanding that you are clear-headed or in recovery now. I have had countless conversations with psychologists and psychiatrists about the delusions I've had. And the more I have these conversations, the more I am able to accept that delusions are a part of my human experience.

I keep the conversation going with my team about my delusions. I tell my friends sometimes. I talk to my family sometimes, although it's not that often. But when I open up, the psychosis becomes a real thing that happened to me, and I can see that it is not inherently who I am. Psychosis is something that around one in 100 people experience. That means I am not alone, and I am not faulty; I have an illness that is a part of my life.

For someone going through psychosis for the first time, you can learn to become aware that the delusions are not your fault, not of your own making. Something is going wrong in your brain. The chemicals are going awry, and it is not shameful or blameworthy. Telling someone relieves a lot of this pressure because you are sharing it and you are not alone with it. When I have told people in the past, their reaction has only been caring. When I am well and I try to detail the delusions I have had, people often can't understand. But if I am in distress and I reach out to anyone, not just those in my team, usually I am met with care. Then the focus turns to getting better. Now, there is a lot that has to happen between these steps, and I am not saying it was or is easy! I just think if there are some small things you can do to alleviate your suffering, not isolating yourself is definitely one of them.

It's true that it has taken me seeing about ten psychiatrists before I found one that I've stuck to, and this isn't because the psychiatrists were bad or I didn't like them. It has to do with the time in my life and my illness. I experienced the worst psychosis of my life in 2018, and it took a lot for me to come back from that. I went to a psychiatrist with community mental health at that time, and I have followed him through telehealth since then. He knows me and has seen my many moves around the country since then. We can pinpoint psychoses and brief episodes (often after the fact). He has helped me keep my recent psychoses mild and brief through monitoring the medication I take. He is also a constant person in my story of schizophrenia, which is important because it has reduced the number of times I have had to go through the story of my illness with each new practitioner. The trauma of repeatedly doing that is awful. Also, having a constant person like that means you build a relationship and you are more likely to trust them in crisis. I have taken my current meds since 2019, and I have confidence in this psychiatrist and the medication he prescribes. It hasn't been without side effects, but it has been with a constant person.

After the psychosis in 2018, I desperately needed to treat my condition with medication, as I had stopped taking it and the result was a disaster. When I look back on that time, I remember I would walk my dog with my earphones in, listening to a song by The Rubens that included the line 'You're the best that there is on this Earth,' and I thought they had written it about me. I must have been getting a lot of dopamine from that belief because it felt good. It was thrilling and exciting. I spent the summer walking my dog and giving away all my possessions out the front of my beach shack up north. I did this in some delusion about not wanting to own anything orange or anything my family had given me or that reminded me of them. I got my personal belongings down to what would fit in a van, and I slept in the van because I thought the beach shack was haunted. I spent Christmas Day on my own, completely enraptured by all these entertaining thoughts. I was going to the doctor but only because I said I had anxiety, so we treated that. This is another example of a time when I could have gotten help earlier but didn't because I didn't disclose my true experience. I had all these hyper-positive feelings from my ideas about being so grandiose. I lied because I liked feeling like that. If you are experiencing feelings like this, the straight and narrow path of "correct" treatment might feel far less appealing than the rush of the high or mania you might feel in psychosis, but that treatment grounds you in reality and you don't do strange things that might embarrass you later.

I didn't have a team around me for the bad psychoses, and I haven't had a bad psychosis since I have had a team around me. That's why I recommend grabbing as many people as you can to be on your team. They can help you. They *want* to help you. You just have to be open to it. As soon as I get any strange thoughts now or I start thinking like I do during a psychosis, I go to the GP. I tell them what is happening. I arrange an appointment with the psychologist or counsellor and sort through it. I go to the psychiatrist and tell them what I am thinking and feeling. This often nips it in the bud. Through these conversations, the people on my team monitor me. We might change the dosage of the medication, or we work through the often anxious thoughts and stress behind the symptoms. Because of this, my psychoses have been less severe, and I have been able to ride them out pretty painlessly. But it has taken a long time to get to this point, and the change for me was gradual.

Sometimes when you are unwell, you can't work or study, but holding on to some purpose and direction in your life through trying to find solutions and get better is so helpful in your recovery. I believe that getting up, getting dressed, and getting out of the house is hugely beneficial for anyone suffering mental illness, and keeping your appointments means you will do this. It offers you a sanity amid the insanity because the reason you are getting up and going out is to see a professional to help you fix a problem you are having. When you get to the appointment, you need to tell the practitioner that you think you might be in a psychosis. Then explain the thoughts or things that make you think this. If you are having suicidal ideation, tell them. This can be confronting, and it might feel like you are giving away your plans and secrets. You might end up going to hospital, but try not to be scared. You are not 'getting locked up.' Rather, you are seeking therapy. These practitioners can access medication and psychology designed to get you well.

The first step is being open to help. Then it's finding the right people. I have been fortunate enough to have benefitted from seeking professional assistance, and I've been able to afford doctor's appointments. Your local doctor should be able help you, so make an appointment and go to it. If you aren't motivated or can't afford to do this, SANE Australia has a free phone line you can call, and community health centres can also provide assistance. If you are uncomfortable with the health professionals you see or if any of your team want to judge you, steer clear. You can also ask someone you love and trust to go to the appointment with you, if possible.

Getting a team around me and keeping my appointments has been a game changer in my journey. I really believe it can make a positive difference for you too.

'The Queen'
There is a Queen among the people.
She is the secret Queen.
She lives a normal life
But is protected by those "in the know."
She gets to experience
Daily life and society's great achievements
As a layperson.
But she's special.
She is also "in the know."
The community does things
To show its excellence,
And she feels grateful and special,
And powerful and royal
She is hidden from foreign countries.
And safe from outside forces.
The secret Queen is the
Main character in the country.
The PM and the people on TV know
All those "in the know."

Chapter 4

Stick to a routine

Routine can be so helpful for anyone experiencing psychosis. This includes things like:
- getting up and going to bed at the same time each day and getting around eight hours' sleep
- brushing your teeth when the day begins and again before bed
- getting dressed
- spiritual practice like prayer and meditation
- exercise
- going out to do something, whether it's an appointment or work
- eating three meals a day
- drinking water.

Sticking to a routine has helped me when I have experienced the cycles of psychosis, and I think I have been able to alleviate the severity of symptoms through maintaining routine errands, tasks and habits.

I always make my bed when I get out of it. This sets my bedroom up for the day and delineates sleep time from daytime. I try to exercise every day; it makes me feel good and happy, and I know it is good for my mental health. I shower, dress, put my make-up on and leave the house with my watch on. I go to work or go out once a day on most days except the weekend. There are rituals in my routine that set me up for the day, make me feel confident, and are special to me. Often, I meditate and pray. These routines help me when I am in psychosis because I am so "in the air" at those times that doing the regular activities of the day helps to ground me, and I can try to relate to reality.

During the years when I first began to experience psychosis, I often drank heavily and did not sleep well. Sometimes I would not brush my teeth, and I would sleep fully clothed. I would sleep during the day and eat poorly. I found reasons to not go out. I would lock myself in my bedroom and hide from the world. Days became nights, and they all mushed into one. I remember not sleeping for a whole night before one of the National Rugby League grand finals, and I was fully immersed in the coverage of the game, which was giving me signs from the conspiracy about my stepdad's life. It was all very strange but felt so natural at the time. I thought there were signs from the universe about racism and about things that were not real, and I sat eating white mayonnaise with white rice crackers in the belief that racism had gotten into my food.

As my life progressed and I got older, my psychoses became a lot more familiar, and I realised that getting routine sleep was a big factor in helping me calm the delusions. Having a solid eight hours of sleep at night has helped me immeasurably, and medication also helps with this. Sleeping, showering, eating three meals a day, brushing my teeth twice a day, going out to work or the shops or the doctor, walking the dog, and showering are all elements of the day that help me in coasting though a psychosis. They keep me in touch with reality and some form of normality, and they help me with understanding what things mean. It's like I tap into a life that existed before the psychoses, and I can touch what it was like then.

I know my schizophrenia has become more manageable since I have stuck to a routine, but I will admit here that I have often gone to work when perhaps I shouldn't have. I turned up and acted normal and pretended I was okay when I wasn't. As much as this was perhaps dangerous and is not recommended, I believe the routine of going to work helped me in getting through certain points. Being at home would have done me more harm. I would go work, often doing minimal duties and sometimes having to go home sick and distressed, sometimes in denial that I was even sick, but always keeping that routine, which I also think helped me build resilience over time. This was because I knew I could still be in public and look fine. I wasn't a total outsider. If I had stayed at home, I would have isolated myself completely, and possibly become a recluse.

I think I have got a lot out of sticking to a routine and going out into the world, even if it was not always the right thing to do. If I had stayed at home as a result of the slightest strange thought, I would never have gone to work and would have lost my career. I pushed through a lot at tough times to keep my job, and as much as I could have done things differently—hindsight is a wonderful thing indeed—I was able to see myself as someone who was employable and someone who could hold on to a job, even if my mind was "broken." Knowing I could still look and act "okay" gave me the confidence to not write myself off as completely disabled in the sense of being unable to perform tasks and losing confidence in my abilities. This self-concept is one thing I am very grateful for and proud of. The fact I still turned up to work might have been necessity, it might have been me in the medical model of disability, it might have been purely economical, but it has helped me come as far as I have today. I have a career, which is one of my greatest assets.

However, it can be hard to create and stick to a routine, especially when you are sick. Little steps help with this. Doing just one thing, like getting out of bed at 7 a.m., can lead to the next thing, but if that feels like it is too much, just get out of bed and make a cup of tea or do something you enjoy. One thing at a time. Break it down into manageable steps when you're starting out, then build things in over time. If you do the routine for a little bit and slip back into old habits, forgive yourself and try again. Start with putting your runners on and walking instead of jogging. Just keep trying. Little steps lead to big gains! The main thing is to be kind to yourself. You've got this.

Make your routine more fun by adding variety from time to time. Change it up. Use a new shampoo, brush your teeth with your non-dominant hand, set your alarm to wake you up with a fun song, walk new routes, sign up for a dance class, or do exercise you like. (I like dancing and rollerblading.) It makes your days much more interesting and enjoyable. You should balance novelty and consistency in your routine and look carefully at what serves you well. Reflect on your routine and look at what works and what does not. Then refine. See how you feel, what is going well and what you could change to make it better.

If you are struggling with your routine, try to remember that even if you don't feel motivated it will help you to feel better and keep a structure in your day. For me, I know it has helped me to stay in touch with the real world by being accountable to my team, and it also gives me confidence when I feel like I am about to crash. Getting dressed and going out, for example, gives me purpose and makes me feel like I did something worthwhile. All my routines that get me out the door when I am feeling good have helped build confidence that I can still go out into the world and perform tasks even when I am unwell. You can do this too.

For more resources, search for "routines" on any of the following organisations' websites.

Verywell Mind
verywellmind.co

ADDitude magazine
additudemag.com

National Institutes of Health (NIH)
ncbi.nim.nih.gov

Beyond Blue
beyondblue.org.au

La Trobe University
latrobe.edu.au

'Okri'
Okri, my pug,
You saw me go mad.
We walked and walked,
And yes, it was bad.
But you stood by me
With your little pig tail,
We walked and walked
In the rain and the hail.
Dear Okri, I'm sorry
I once ran away.
I drove the van south
And left you to stay.
I came to myself
Somewhere on the Hume.
I had to ring Lisa

To go and get you.
I left you alone.
In the beach shack
With water and snack
And didn't come back.

Chapter 5

Quit the drugs, cigarettes and alcohol

Another piece of my experience, and what I think helps a great deal in surviving psychosis, is quitting drugs, cigarettes and alcohol. And as with the suggestions given in previous chapters, this is easier said than done, but the benefits are astounding.

It is estimated 50% of people with schizophrenia have a history of substance abuse (www.addictioncenter.com/addiction/schizophrenia). I think this is often a case of self-medicating or trying to relieve symptoms. This statistic means we are often afflicted with both our illness and the side effects of using any of these substances, and this makes our health outcomes poorer than the general population. I think it sucks. I want to see people with psychosis kicking goals, not going into hospital for lung cancer or liver disease.

Using drugs, cigarettes and alcohol is often a self-soothing behaviour for those of us with schizophrenia I know I used them for a long time to medicate my delusions. I also wanted to fit in and be cool with my peers before I had my first psychosis. Trying to escape myself was something that I seemed to like A LOT. Then I used these substances to try to escape my mind. I couldn't understand what was going on, so I drank it away. I would be going at a hundred miles an hour mentally, and the booze would slow it all down. I have an addictive personality, so complete abstinence has worked for me. But if you are overusing any of these substances to medicate yourself, perhaps moderation might help you.

I'll tell you my experience, starting with drugs. I took drugs as a young person, and I believe that this is one of the reasons that I suffer this illness today, although it's true that my friends who took drugs at the same time and with same level of consumption as me did not experience what I have. They do not have a chronic mental illness now. But without knowing the possible consequences, I took drugs as a young person, and I found them very alluring and fun. I felt free and excited when I was on them, but often I would also feel paranoid and scared. I thought it was cool to take drugs. That's why I did it. I wanted to fit in and be one of the group.

I sniffed things, took tablets and inhaled the burnt embers of green stuff. My friends and I wagged school, went to festivals and drove to the river where we would do the drugs. It seemed daring and illicit. I loved the rush. At one festival, I took my pill early in the afternoon and "peaked" when I felt the big rush of serotonin get released in my brain. Then I spent the rest of the night in the car, scared and paranoid that my friends were laughing at me, fearful for my life. It was horrible. The high was never worth the comedown. I would smoke pot in my bedroom and write in my diary and draw. Then the next day, I would think everyone was talking about me at school. It was intense—so intense that after I was in hospital that first time for psychosis, I knew I needed to stop taking drugs. They made everything so much harder. I would think strange things and get super paranoid. I knew I needed to not smoke pot at least. It was so bad for my brain, and my time in hospital was the wake-up call I needed. So, I stopped smoking pot altogether.

The next thing I managed to quit was smoking. I was a heavy smoker. I would go for a jog and come home and have a ciggie. I loved it. I was addicted. I would have one with my morning coffee. I would have one when I was bored. I would have one when I had a break at work. I would have one after a hard day. I loved the nicotine hit. I got pleasure out of that little bit of dopamine. I got a rush because it was a "treat" that didn't have calories. Smoking was glamourous, or so I thought, and I wanted to look pained chic, like Angelina Jolie's character in *Girl Interrupted*. Oh dear. What this led to was 16 years of sucking smoke into my precious lungs. Yuck! As a result, I was never really fit enough when I played sport or jogged, which made me feel bad all the time. I always had to go outside and be removed from whatever situation I was in because I wanted to smoke. I was never present or connected to anyone because I was always thinking about my next cigarette. I wanted to quit, but I couldn't find the resources or willpower to do it. I tried countless times, but it never worked. I have hundreds of diaries entries encouraging myself to quit. I beat myself up constantly. I loved smoking, but I also absolutely detested it.

Finally, I bought a book that said it would help me quit: Allen Carr's *Easyway to Quit Smoking*. I read it once, and I started smoking again. But the second time I read it, I got it. I stopped. And I stayed stopped. The key thing I took from that book was that it wasn't painful to quit, that there was no pain involved. I read about addiction, and I read about the fact that I would put down my last cigarette, and I did. I have never looked back. I kept drinking, but I stopped smoking. That meant I could get fit. I could breathe freely. I could smell good. In fact, I soon felt sick when I smelt someone smoking a cigarette. This made me feel good. I became disgusted by smoking. I was a non-smoker, and it was delightful!

There are still times when I think I could take it up again and have a calorie-free dopamine hit, but I resist the urge and I talk to people about it. No one ever regrets quitting smoking. I think about my health, the money I have saved and all the freedom I have now that I am not an addict. It is truly wonderful!

Let's look now at the drinking. I went from teenage years through my twenties still smoking cigarettes and drinking A LOT. I couldn't see a life without drinking; it was ingrained in the culture around me. All my friends and family drank, and there was a huge party lifestyle at university and in my early teaching career. My friends and I would get together for Friday night drinks, which would extend to after-sport drinks on Saturday and sometimes also a "Sunday session" on Sunday after-noons. These weekends often saw me blacking out and doing things I regretted. I would proposition men and women for sex, sleep with them, vomit, dance crazily and be vile, causing all sorts of drama. I had a good time, don't get me wrong, but I would spend the better part of the next week getting over it. I would have to work out what had happened, apologise to people and sometimes get tests for sexually transmitted diseases. I would rumi-nate on things, blowing them out of proportion, fearing what I had done. I would experience intense shame and horror over my actions on the weekend nights. These were huge things for a young person to deal with, espe-cially someone who was starting a career and trying to find their way in the world with a mental illness.

Over time, I began to medicate the psychosis with alcohol. I would go into the strange thoughts, thinking people had secret messages to share with me through code, then get home and down half a cask of cheap sauvignon blanc to erase the memories, to stop the thought train, to ease the pain. I would obliterate myself on weeknights, passing out and then getting up and going to work in the morning. I stayed in this cycle for a long time.

During my first teaching post, I had psychosis and was so ashamed I drank it away. I was so fearful I might be different or faulty that I played the party girl. I had other teachers comment about my drinking. I got asked to turn off the music on weeknights in the teacher accommodation where I lived, and I was so alone with the battle in my mind. I decided to change schools and move to a farmhouse out of town where I could play my music really loud and drink as much as I wanted and not have to answer to anyone. What a terrible decision! What a terrible time. At this point, I became dependent on alcohol. I emailed my superiors while I was drunk at home, sending them random things like song lyrics or philosophical rants that were nonsense. The alcohol-fuelled psychosis got out of control. Other teachers had me on suicide watch. My mum came out to the farm to try to get me medicated and get me home. I refused. I thought she was evil, and I pretended I was okay, not giving in to her requests. She said, 'Poppy, the principal has called me. They are worried about you.' I laughed in her face and said I was fine. By now, I was on special leave from work, drinking and being hungover most of the time. It took being cut from the special leave program and having my pay cut for me to wake up. I had run out of options. I was at the end. I had to move home.

Obligingly, I went to a psychiatrist, got medicated, moved back to Mum's and got a job in a factory. I was gutted. I thought I had completely failed. I was so ashamed and self-conscious. I believed those emails to the boss were a part of who I was. I didn't realise I had a chronic illness and was medicating it. I saw myself as being faulty, making up for my sins. I was so desperate to not be seen as sick, and I thought I could drink normally.

Believe it or not, my drinking career continued for another six years, only I binged rather than drank every day because I believed I had "learnt my lesson" from my time at the farmhouse. I thought sorting cow lungs on the factory conveyor belt was my punishment for what had happened. I didn't deserve to be a teacher after what I had done. I felt terrible. Around this time, everyone I knew was getting married, buying homes and having kids, and here I was, living with my parents and trying not spew on the cow lungs. This was a really hard time.

It took a few years for me to get the guts to get back into the teaching the game. I was over the menial tasks I was doing in my other jobs, and I wanted to do something more meaningful. I was exercising and looking to the future. It took a while, but I felt stronger and ready to give my career another crack after being on medication for four years. I moved to my aunt's place in a different town and got a teaching gig again. I drank only on the weekends, when I would ramble crap and whinge and bitch about everyone getting married. I caused a lot of drama for my aunt and the people I met. I was battling. I had another psychosis and left town again, this time moving up north to the coast. I still thought drinking was okay for me, and I still took my meds. Until I wanted to lose weight. I wanted to look great, like the surfer chicks, so I began losing weight very dramatically.

One night, drank very heavily. I was so drunk my friend got angry and left me at the pub, where I was adamant that I was having more fun than anyone else. The pub closed, and I walked back to my friend's place and got in the car to drive the five-minute journey home. But I don't remember this. What I remember is the blue lights flashing in my rear-view mirror. I remember not being able to blow hard enough into the breathalyser because I was too intoxicated. I remember crying to the police officers that I was a teacher and I couldn't have a criminal record. I woke up with the ticket on my bedside table and no car and no licence. This was my new hell. I had to call Mum. I had to call my head teacher. I had to call my friends to help me get my car. I called a close friend, who told me I should join a 12-step program. I made the call that day, and I haven't had a drink since.

I could have killed someone that night. I could have killed myself. I am so grateful I was pulled over and stopped by the police. I am so glad I got that wake-up call. Even so, the ensuing months were awful. I walked to school, and the students knew why. I was alone and scared and ashamed, and I had the worst psychosis of my life. This is when I thought I was the secret Queen with the ticket for driving under the influence of alcohol. The TV was talking to me, and my delusions were so wild I think they were the only way I could experience pleasure at this time in my life. I was going to the doctor but not to treat the psychosis. I was treating my broken heart and my anxiety. It was all very confusing!

I spent a lot of time not drinking without any support, and it was really hard. I rejoined the 12-step fellowship a year or so later, and I was able to connect with other people who had drinking problems. This has been a total blessing. As a result of not drinking, I have been able to ward off intense psychoses earlier, and I have FAR LESS drama in my life. I don't have guilt, shame and remorse for days on end after drinking. I will never drink drive again. I don't have to worry about what I might do or say when drunk because I simply don't pick up the first drink. Most importantly, I don't *need* to drink anymore. This has been a revelation for me. I never believed I would be able to quit drinking. I went on dry months or said I wouldn't drink for a weekend, but I always went back. It was a never-ending cycle that I was using to medicate myself, but it actually exacerbated everything in my life and made it about fifty times worse!

I am so glad I am a non-drinker now. Instead of drinking, I spend my time trying to be present and spiritual. I write and read and go to the gym, with no need to go to Friday night drinks and wipe myself out or prove anything to anyone. I am me. I don't drink, and I understand that I need to be sober for my mental health. Since quitting drinking, I have only had that one big psychosis immediately afterward and a few brief reactive ones in the years since. I have done all the things that I recommend in this book, and they have made all the difference.

If you or someone you know is trying to quit anything, I say never give up on giving up! Keep trying, because one day the penny will drop. I have seen it dozens of times with people I know who have wanted to quit and not gotten there the first time. That's okay. Keep trying. Joining that 12-step fellowship worked for me, and I believe this is a good resource if you need it, but there are others too. Community mental health and your GP can help you to quit. Alcoholics Anonymous, Narcotics Anonymous, Sober in the Country and the Quitline in Australia are all great resources too.

Let's kick the drugs, kick the smokes and kick the booze so we can start kicking those life goals instead.

'Dear Alcohol'
You gave me confidence
And took me out of my head.
I bid goodbye to booze
And I found God instead.

In the car, I tried to drive,
Should have ended up dead.
I bid goodbye to booze
And I found God instead.

Getting sober it was hard,
From sanity I fled.
I bid goodbye to booze
And I found God instead.

Spirit Universe is my God,
Not Jesus who bled.
I bid goodbye to booze
And I found God instead.

Recovering, I am alive,
Sheets of trauma I have shed.
I bid goodbye to booze
And I found God instead.

Content and happy I am now,
And stable on my meds.
I bid goodbye to booze
And I found God instead.

Chapter 6

Express yourself creatively

Expressing yourself creatively is important for people who experience psychosis, as it is for all human beings. Whether it's writing, singing, dancing, playing an instrument, knitting, drawing, painting, designing things, or engaging in in some other creative endeavour, there is a lot to be said for art therapy. Art therapy is a healing strategy that can improve wellbeing.

A few days into my first hospital admission in 2005, I was led to a room and given some paint and paper and told to explore what I was feeling. It wasn't a proper class, and I didn't know what to do, but with all the chaos going on in my head, all the worrying I was doing about what people thought of me, all the delusions and the trauma I was going through, I found that applying the liquid paint onto the paper put me into the moment and made my mind still for a time. I only made blobs of paint on the paper that day, but the peace that this brought me was precious. And from then on, I knew that creative outlets were important.

My most recent psychosis saw me write my way through it. I didn't write down the delusions as I had them, but I commented on things that I thought about as if I were a writer, as if it mattered. I wrote about my past, about teaching, about the environment, about travelling and philosophy. I wrote poems about my sexuality and penned letters to the paper about recycling organic waste. These were all ways I was expressing myself and helping to make sense of my very unstable and tumultuous inner world. It was using my lexicon to create something that didn't exist before. It was not a waste of time; it held purpose in keeping me on track, giving me an outlet after work and using that agreed upon code, which is language, to help me make sense of reality.

Here's a poem I wrote during that time about my addiction to social media.

'Screen Sucking'
I can't stop the screen sucking me in,
Makes me flighty,
Plays with my thoughts.
Colours and images, bright and happy,
Not reality, where I reside.

Things aren't always like those images.

There's a lot of boring and banal,
Gross and painful,
Screen sucking my eyes.

Then I pat my dog or make a fire
And I return to Earth, to primal,
So authentically natural and real.
Breath and now, here it is.

I am sucking the screen
For a shiny illusion, an idea,
Constant. Open the app/close the app,
Open it again without realising,

Scoping for new content, for something,
I don't know what.
The black craving ghost
Lives within.

The screen sucks me into ideas about
Myself, what I could be,
What I'm not,
What I plan to do.

Sucking screen vacuums my soul,
And that fire and my dog
Are secondary
To the world of the internet.

And among all the people online,
I am alone
Under the stars,
Staring at the sucking screen.

The desire to share everything,
To represent myself,
To express my excitement
Has been monetised.

Apps make me the product
And the consumer at once,
Infiltrating all my experiences.
'How will I caption this?'

I want to keep the moment;
I want to share the moment.
My love for things is intertwined
With the sucking screen.

It's never a bad thing to express yourself. Even if no one sees it, even if no one likes it. It helps you to process what is happening. Creativity is a vital part of being a human, and it helps with mental health so much.

Throughout my life, I have kept a diary. This has helped me define reality and process things through all kinds of trauma in my life. Sexual assault as a child, break-ups with boyfriends, sex, quitting alcohol and trying to understand myself are all things I have processed through writing. I have about 70 diaries that I've kept since I was eight years old. These diaries have travelled with me over 15 house moves and many crazy psychoses. Once, I drove five hours to steal them from where they were being kept in my parents' rumpus room because I thought my parents might read them. The diaries are hilarious and heartbreaking. Some of them make me want to go back in time and hug the girl who was writing those words. Others contain many, many false promises about tomorrow being the day I quit smoking, lose weight and stop drinking forever. Over and over again, I would repeat myself. The diaries are boring in many places. They are banal and repetitive. But much as I labelled those promises as false after the fact, they were all part of my process. And being able to go back and read that process, to be able to see it in front of me—even my writer's voice has completely transformed with age—is a wonderful thing.

I always wanted to be creative and make my mark on the world. I had ambitions to become an actress and a writer, but I got really busy with trying to survive. Looking back on my creative outpourings, I am astounded I was resilient in times of pure horror, and I am so proud of that. This makes me want to express myself even more! I especially love that I write. I am a solo traveller, and I don't have a partner, so writing also helps me to remember and share things from my journeys. I haven't gotten too far in finding an audience for my writing, but I have sent some articles away for publication in local women's journals. Some of my letters to the editor have been published, and I have given love poems to partners. I also reckon that one day I will publish a memoir from my 32-odd years of journalling.

Contrary to my poem above, social media is another great outlet for me to express myself, even if in a contained and sanitary way. I love sharing the good bits of my life because I am so grateful for them. I have stopped caring whether I look like I am bragging all the time or whether I am oversharing on social media accounts. I am simply so enamoured with the things I get to do and have and experience when I am not simply surviving psychosis. I post about my camping and the adventures I go on and the things I do on the weekend and the things I am grateful for. People press like on these posts or comment that it looks like I'm having fun. I like this positive feedback. It makes me feel good. It reinforces that I am well and that I am doing well.

It is a bit of a stereotype to say a lot of great art was created by people who were mentally ill, but it has definitely helped me on my journey. My advice is to try different ways of expressing yourself creatively, whether it is something you liked doing when you were younger or something totally new to you. Choose something and have a go. Have fun. Play. Engage in the moment and enjoy the process. Creativity takes you away from the really hard stuff that life can throw at you, and it allows you to process those difficult emotions that can come up.

Schizy Inc in Melbourne has great creative workshops, such as drama and acting, writing and artmaking, for people with complex mental illness. The Dax Centre is another place where you can learn about creative expression—both your own and that of other people with lived experience of mental illness.

Creativity can be purely personal, but you can also become a part of a community who all engage in the art. That can lead to all kinds of friendships and collaborative projects as well, so start exploring possibilities!

'Express'
My only way of processing
Is to write.
I adore it.
I love it.
Creative expression is
Life-affirming,
Exciting, bubbly, ethereal.
I can't help that I want
To tell my story.
Here I am.
This is me.
I want to express myself
And be proud.
I want to tell stories.
I love stories,
I love through stories.
I live stories,

I live through stories.
Expression is delight,
Like the first coffee of the day.
Expression is colour,
Like a gouache painting.
Living and loving,

Chapter 7

Exercise

The Zumba class is full. We are midway through Ricky Martin's 'She Bangs,' we are jumping, smiling, sweaty. We move in unison. The instructor is jumping too, a bit better than us. Our hands are in the air. Our feet are stepping and jumping about. The music is loud, I am sweaty and delighted, a big silly grin on my face because I feel alive, strong and confident. I feel the blood rushing around my body with my breath. To move is to feel free. Ecstatic, we sing along and express ourselves rhythmically. I love it!

I know it gets drummed into you by all the doctors and all the health professionals, but exercise is VITAL, and it makes *you* vital. I believe exercise is one of the main methods by which I have been able to manage my psychosis in a relatively logical way. When I say logical, I mean I put exercise into the routine I spoke about before and I use it as a ritual to practice mindfulness and determination. Exercise has made me stronger physically and mentally. It can be compared to creativity as an outlet, and I say this because you can get creative with it, and you can experience the same kind of satisfaction from exercise as you get when you are creative.

When I exercise, I feel my body come alive. I use it to celebrate what my body can do. When I was younger, exercise was all about losing weight and looking a certain way, but now it is a feelgood activity to boost my well-being. It gives me those nice feelings in my brain and body that I used to get with the first couple of drinks. Dopamine, I believe it is. Exercise also gives me confidence in my body, that I can do things and feel my muscles working, even though I don't work excessively hard while exercising. I tend to lift the same amount of weight and follow the same route on my jog. I don't continually seek improvement. I exercise for the feeling it gives me and for the celebration of my body, and I believe this is a healthy way to view it, not doing it to punish myself or constantly push myself but moving simply to feel good. Feeling joy and pleasure in your body is one of life's great gifts, I have found.

Once again, it's easier said than done, and exercise needs to be done in a healthy way. When I had my first psychosis, I decided to jog instead of taking my meds. This is an example of an unhealthy way of using exercise to survive psychosis. As I have grown older and weathered the storms of countless psychoses, I have found exercise to be a wonderful way to help me cope and manage. My psychosis of 2018 saw me walking my dog every day, mainly because I wanted the dog to be healthy and get to sniff all the smells! But this also got me out of the house. It gave me fresh air, raised my heart rate and gave me good endorphins that helped my brain. I wasn't a danger to myself or anyone else by doing this. I rode out the psychosis safely until I realised I was sick and needed to get help. But those walks helped me. I don't know much about the science of exercise. I can only speak from experience and common knowledge, but that routine, rain, hail or shine, made me feel good and kept me feeling healthy.

Over time, I have found ways to enjoy exercise more. I use it to blow off steam by taking boxing classes. I use it to laugh, joke and have fun by taking Zumba classes. I use it to fit in and make friends by playing in a soccer team. I use it to be present and practise meditation and breathwork by swimming and jogging. I absolutely love doing these things, but there are always moments and challenges, like when my mind wanders into regrets and doubt in the pool or when I feel like I am the worst player on the soccer team. These things are minor setbacks, however, when I weigh up the benefits I experience from my exercise. I have learnt to celebrate what my body can do, not what it looks like. This was a big lesson for me. I haven't needed the "thin and fit" success story to feel good about myself; success is now on my own terms.

In Osher Gunsberg's book *Back, After the Break*, he writes about getting into exercise to manage his mental health. He got out of the house and walked the block, repeating the route until he wanted to walk for longer. So, he went a bit longer, and then his walks turned into jogging. I have done the same thing as Osher, although my jogging is more of shuffle alongside my dog, who is old and slow. I don't do it to compete or to keep to that linear story of constant improvement. I do it to see the sunrise and to breathe the morning air deeply into my lungs. I do it for my dog, and you can find a reason to do it too. Just walk a little bit to start with or lift a really light weight. Show up to the dance class or the yoga class or the gym, and be prepared to be a beginner. You might just love it. You might start to feel strong and more confident like me. You might not. I just know it has helped me so much over the years, and I recommend that you try it.

However, exercise might not be as beneficial or straightforward for everyone as it has been for me. People who have severe eating disorders or who have had bad experiences in the past might not like it the way I do, and that is okay. But looking after your body is important, and I encourage you to find some way to move yours that is healthy and enjoyable. You can care for your body in other ways too, like having a bath or putting on moisturiser. Having rituals that enable you to enjoy your body and experience pleasure from it will make you feel good and boost your wellbeing. Exercising with a friend is fun too. They might be a part of your team and help to motivate you. Your body is precious, so treat it well. You are worth it.

'My Body'
I want to celebrate
What my body can do
Rather than punish it
For what how it looks.
My body is sacred
And what it does for me
Is endless wonder
Care-fully.

Chapter 8

Share your story

Sharing your story with others, through web forums, social media, creative expression or in support groups, is another piece of advice that I believe has helped me with my management of psychosis. Telling people about your experience reduces stigma and helps you to understand the reality of it. It also opens doors to communication and the sharing of ideas about what happened, what helps, and how you can deal with things.

I have been an avid anonymous contributor to the SANE forum since 2016. I have written there many times to share my story and to communicate my lived experience. I have found that this is a safe space where I can whinge about the stigma I have faced. Sharing your story is not always safe, however. I have tried to do this in a professional context, and it has been a disaster!

When I was reapplying for permanency in the teaching profession, there was a box to tick on the form about pre-existing medical conditions. I stressed for days about answering this question. I didn't know what to write. I thought the employer might have a file on me about the time I went on special leave or records about my psychosis from when I was previously employed. I didn't want them to think I was lying if ticked no. I agonised over what to do, and in the end, I ticked yes and wrote schizophrenia next to it. I sent the forms off.

It took the employer six weeks to get back to me. They wanted letters from my psychiatrist saying I was fit to work. The process dragged on for another six months. Apparently, the employer went to my principal and asked personal questions about me. I was trying to work out whether this was discrimination or not and what would have happened if I had just ticked no instead of yes. Somehow or another, I redid the forms at another point when trying to find a permanent job. This time, I ticked no to having a medical condition and never admitted anything. I got the job.

I think this says a lot about disability discrimination in organisations. It also shows there is a massive stigma toward the word "schizophrenia." It was 2018 when I filled in those forms. We have come a long way since then, although there is a lot more progress yet to be made. Neurodiversity is seen as more normalised now, and things are moving along in terms of employment for people with disabilities. My employer has targets for people identifying as having a disability to be employed with them. The media has also come a long way in its portrayal of schizophrenia. There is less emphasis on people with schizophrenia being criminal, "crazy" or "psycho," and it is seen as more of disability than a disease that serial killers have.

I shared on the SANE forum the story about my employer and what happened when I ticked the box for yes. It is a public forum, so anyone can read that post. I believe sharing this story has contributed to the shift in attitude in society. I have shared much of my story anonymously, and I hope it has helped others. The more awareness and conversations we have around complex mental health, the better. It means people can get help quicker, and there isn't all that shame tied into it when you realise something is wrong. The stigma is so much less now than it once was, but we still have a long way to go. More ethical and equitable processes and better access for people with disability; more open mindedness from people, particularly employers; and greater education about people with disability *by* people with disability are some of the things I think we could do better.

Telling people about psychosis can be quite tricky. I say "tricky" because it's such a complex thing it can be difficult to describe. Saying the words 'I get psychosis' is a good place to start, but often people want to know more. It is hard for them to understand. I have told people I thought I was the Queen of Australia, and they were flabbergasted. 'How can that be? How does that work? Were you on drugs?' Then I have to explain the intricacies. 'No, I wasn't on drugs. This is something that happens to me regularly, and I take a heavy dose of medication for it.'

Because there are still a lot of unknowns about psychosis in the medical profession, it is hard to pinpoint the cause of it. I say that I have a chemical imbalance in my brain and that I need to rebalance it with medication. I say that the psychosis might be because I took drugs when I was young or it might be because I might have a predisposition towards it from my family. The situation is so unclear to me, so trying to make it clear to someone else is hard, but I like being honest with people. I like sharing my story because the person I share it with now knows someone with schizophrenia and that means it becomes less distant and scary to them. Sharing our stories brings more familiarity about the topic, and it encourages people to try to understand it more. They can say they know someone with psychosis when they are talking about it to others, and that builds more knowledge and helps to conquer the fear around it.

I have shared my story countless times, and I have never really had a horrible reaction to it, although sometimes I need to go deeper to try to get the listener to understand. Some people find it really hard to believe. This can be hurtful, like I have to justify myself and my experience to them. I think people with invisible disabilities and mental illness have always battled this kind of disbelief, but most people care when you tell them, and they want to know more. They want to know how they can help, and they are sometimes fascinated and admiring of what you have been through.

Telling different people can mean telling your story in different ways. For example, telling a new GP about your experience with psychosis is vastly different to telling a new love interest. A good GP will ask for a bit of history and how you manage it. A good love interest will be concerned with helping you. But that's not always the case. I have had love interests blame my bad moods or arguments on my illness. I have had GPs not believe I am unwell because I am a teacher and I finished a degree. People have different opinions and reactions, and that's their thing. It's not yours. Your disclosing is a gift to them, and if their reaction is poor, you might have to find someone else to tell.

One time, I needed to share my story and didn't. I was in the principal's office at the school where I worked, and they were concerned about me. I had gone quiet and was acting detached. The kids' learning was suffering. I didn't share my story on this occasion, and I deeply regret it. I was so sick and full of denial and shame that I could not speak. If I had shared my story at this time, it would have been met with support and I would not have had to resign. Instead, I kept quiet and walked out, blaming the principal for thinking I was sick. This was a huge lesson for me. Sharing your story can be scary, but it can also be so important at critical times.

Share your story when you need to, when life-changing situations arise and when you feel safe to do so. Be careful of stigma, and if your story is not accepted by the people you tell, find others who will listen to what you say and respond with compassion and understanding.

Here are some places where you can find support and share your story.

One Door

onedoor.org.au

SANE Australia

sane.org

Uniting has a program in Melbourne and Ballarat called Hearing Voices

unitingvictas.org.au/services/mental-health/hearing-voices-support

'My Alternative Identity'

I am an advocate for schizophrenia,

Going on the telly

And stuff like that.

We aren't murderers and terrorists,

I'll show them,

Instead of hiding from everyone,

Fear of stigma

Of getting the sack.

I'll be selling my memoir and be famous,

A writer, an activist,

That is me.

My alternative identity.

Chapter 9

Advocate, smash stigma and participate!

My next piece of advice is something I am only just learning, and it has taken me many years to get to this point. I have never been public with my illness, except once saying on Facebook that I'd I had a breakdown. That was one of those confessional-type posts that everyone was supportive about. I was grateful for that, but I have been holding off on stating my diagnosis explicitly until now. I have never directly addressed psychosis or schizophrenia anywhere in public with my name on it. I don't know if people have been ready to hear it. I know in my workplace they haven't.

When it comes to advocacy and smashing stigma, I have been inspired by appearance activist Carly Findlay in her work about disability and by Heidi Everett and Sandy Jeffs in their work on schizophrenia. Both Carly and Sandy have been awarded Medals of the Order of Australia for their advocacy and activism in the disability community, and both have appeared in episodes of the ABC TV show *You Can't Ask That*. Sandy is a poet who found hope in the fact that she could say she is a poet instead of saying she is schizophrenic. She has written several books about her illness. Heidi is another a poet and writer, and she works with Schizy Inc in Melbourne. These three women have shown me that having disability and being in the public eye can be so helpful for others. I know seeing Carly, Heidi and Sandy in the public eye has helped me feel less shame, less alone and proud of my achievements.

Public advocacy is not for everyone, but advocating for yourself is! Ask for what you need. Seek help. And if you want to advocate for others too, do it because it is SO helpful. I know how much shame and fear I have felt over the years. People who speak up and show their pride in the social domain have inspired me and given me strength many times. Seeing and hearing them, I don't feel so alone. I feel strength and pride. This is where I am up to in my life and my story. I am almost ready to take the leap into the public eye. By publishing this book, I am doing just that.

Another thing I have recently done is to attend forums and workshops put on by organisations like SANE Australia, Beyond Blue, the Black Dog Institute, Schizy

Inc, Headspace and Lifeline, who have members with lived experience of schizophrenia. This has helped me be inspired by others, and it gives us a platform to speak about things like the social model of disability, issues facing people with complex mental health issues, and initiatives and government projects. I have benefited from all of these things immeasurably in my identity and acceptance of my illness.

Coming together and connecting through organisations and forums like these empowers us to smash stigma, which is another way we can all help each other. There is a StigmaWatch program run by SANE Australia that helps people who are facing stigma in big organisations and industries such as the media. Just by being yourself, you are smashing stigma. We are not all serial killers like the stereotype would have us be. We are not all violent like the media sometimes says we are. We are smashing stigma by being ourselves and living our lives, and our allies can help us with smashing stigma and being ourselves living our lives. Our advocates can help us with smashing stigma and being ourselves and living our lives.

Politics and policies play a big role in our lives, and we can advocate and participate in these areas too. We can lobby governments for better mental health services. We can write letters, protest and speak to our local MPs. Maybe someone you know might like to help you pen a letter to a government minister or to your local council, telling of your experience of the mental health system and what you think would help you and others like you. Someone else might advocate for you if they think the system needs change or repair and you're not able to take on the task yourself.

I also want to recommend that you participate in research and studies. Of course, these studies need to be ethical and run by accredited universities or institutions, but this is another way we can help each other and make connections. We need to create communities of people who suffer this illness so we know we are not alone, and this is another way we can help our fellow sufferers and build the body of knowledge about schizophrenia.

We must be strong and stand up for ourselves and our communities when we are well enough to do so. I think I am ready now, but not everyone is at this same place with their illness. That is okay. There are a lot of ways in which we can support and protect each other, and helping others is a wonderful way to take your mind off your own plight, I have found. Helping others and serving the community is a great way to feel good and have a sense of purpose. I wholeheartedly recommend that you get involved!

'Love and Psychosis'
I want you, dear future partner,
To know my past,
To unpack the trauma and sit with me.

Sip tea and understand, dear parents,

It wasn't your fault.
I am here,
Recovering.

At a party for my 40th, dear siblings,
I thank you for your support.
You've seen me
Terrible.

Dear nieces and nephew,

And, my dear students, one day
You will read this and know
I was psychotic once, but
Recovering now

Today celebrate my success, dear friends,
And appreciate, and
Smash stigma
With others.

Growing older, we all are
Love.

From Poppy.

Chapter 10

Practise gratitude

Today's gratitude list looks like this. I am grateful for:
My sobriety
My mental health
Soda water
A text from a love interest
Working hard
Swimming with my nieces
Coffee
A phone call with a friend.

Hugh Van Cuylenburg in his book *The Resilience Project* endorses gratitude. My 12-step fellowship does too. The Dalai Lama talks about it. Most self-help gurus promote it. Why? Because it works! We all have blessings and things that happen throughout the day that are good. Reflecting on these at the end of the day is transformative. I am a happier person now than I have ever been before because I count my blessings and share them with a group of women every day. I highlight what I love about my life, and I take note of good things when they happen. I pay attention, and I feel thankful. Each of the women in the group writes a list of around ten things we're grateful for, and we text message these lists each other. We press the like button on each other's lists to show we've read them. Not only do I feel heard when someone reads my list, but I also feel a warm feeling in my belly because I read over my list at night before I go to sleep, and I feel good about my day and my life. We get specific in what we write, for example we write details of conversations or small moments, and we try to vary what we write for our gratitude so we don't bore each other with the same things every night. This whole practice has been life-changing for me.

Ask someone you know if you can share gratitude lists with each other every day to see if it improves your outlook. Try if for ten days. Swap lists with someone so you can follow and support and applaud one another. I guarantee you will be surprised at the good things you can find! Sometimes it may be very difficult to find things to be grateful for. In these instances, I suggest coming back to your breath and looking for small positives to embrace. They can be moment to moment. You don't always have to write it down, either. Gratitude can be to the Spirit or the Universe and can be said in prayer. Gratitude can be thanking someone you reach out to for help.

I have found that gratitude has made me highlight why I am lucky. I find those things in my life that are precious and sacred, and this has helped me get stronger in building my personal grit.

'Gratitude'
Breath by breath,
I am humble
And crazily in love
With the day.

Soda water and how
You like fungi,
And that song
In the car.

Sunlight on diamond grass.
Cool mornings.
Flannelette.
Brown crunchy leaves.

Swims, all the swims!
A smile, a smell.
Cool aunty vibes.
Fairy bread.

Learning a lesson,
Catching up on things.
Grapefruit.

Earrings.

Pink and orange together.
Anticipation.
Succulents.
Clutter, your clutter.

Op shops and halloumi.
Connection and love.
All the potential.
Thank you.

Afterword

All the advice I've offered you in this book is what I have discovered has worked for me over many years of living with psychosis. It involved a lot of painful trial and error and mistake-making that has seen me learn what I think I can pass on to you. I have felt so much shame and a lack of belonging for so long, and what I want you to know is that *you are not alone*. You are one of many people with this illness, and anyone who experiences it knows how hard it is! I wish I had a book like this when I was in my twenties, with ideas to help me get through psychosis from someone who had experience with it. That is why I have written this: to tell my story, but also to help people like you.

I hope this book has provided you with some practical tools. Telling someone, taking your meds, getting a team around you and keeping your appointments, sticking to a routine, quitting harmful and addictive substances, expressing yourself creatively, exercising, sharing your story, getting active in advocating and smashing stigma, and practising gratitude have all helped me on my very rocky but very worthwhile journey through schizophrenia thus far. I am grateful to have an able body and to have medication that works for me. I am lucky to have a job and to have obtained a degree. My current job involves helping high school students with disability, and it ties in perfectly with the advocacy that is the next step on my journey.

I wish you well, and I hope you get one or two pieces of advice from this book that make you think you are awesome to live through this confusing and terrible illness. Let's engage with the community of folk who live with this. Let's let people know about psychosis, and let's do our best—whatever our best is at the time—to live to our potential. I implore you to be proud and enjoy things in your life.

We can learn to survive psychosis and learn to live well with it.